# 10-Day Green Smoothie Cleanse and + 50 Green Smoothie Recipes for Losing Weight

# By Rebecca Publishing

10-Day Green Smoothie Cleanse and + 50 Green Smoothie Recipes for Losing Weight By Rebecca Publishing

## *Disclaimer*

All the material contained in this book is provided for informational and educational purposes only. No responsibility can be taken for any outcomes resulting from the use of this material.

While every attempt has been made to provide information that is both accurate and effective, the author does not assume any responsibility for the accuracy or use/misuse of this information.

## *About the author!*

Hello my dear readers, I have a lot of information to tell you. I have been studying healthy way of eating from leading nutritionist in Europe and I have a lot of useful information on this topic. I have lost more than 20 kilos so I can provide you with a lot of practical tips on this matter.

My story is also very bright, after giving birth to a child; I have gained a lot of extra weight. It was simply impossible to look into the mirror, but I decided to do my best to return to my previous shape. I have tried swimming, jogging, different diets like Dukan, Sugar Free Diet, Kremlyovskaya Diet etc. These diets forced me to starving and nothing more. I saw and fell the best result after following the Paleo Diet combining with Green Smoothie Cleanse. This diet helped me to loose ALL my extra weight this is more than 20 kilos/44 pounds and I feel myself much healthier now! So, I am glad to share with you 50 of my beloved Green Smoothie Cleanse Recipes, I hope you will find them healthy and delicious as well.

## *Introduction*

Thank you for downloading of my manual: 10-Day Green Smoothie Cleanse and + 50 Green Smoothie Recipes for Losing Weight. All the recipes were tried and prepared by me and they really helped me to loose weight and stay healthy at the same time. I am more than happy to share them with you! You will find a lot of really useful information in this book, they are the following:

- Main facts about Green Smoothies

- Main facts about which foods to avoid

- Main facts about which foods to eat

- Why should we choose Greens?

- Great variety of Green Smoothies for your health

- And 50 amazing Green Smoothie Recipes

# 10-Day Green Smoothie Cleanse and + 50 Green Smoothie Recipes for Losing Weight By Rebecca Publishing

## *The contents*

# 10-Day Green Smoothie Cleanse and + 50 Green Smoothie Recipes for Losing Weight By Rebecca Publishing

### *10-Day Green Smoothie Cleanse important information*

A huge number of people in the world suffer from obesity, various diseases caused by unhealthy diet and lifestyle. We are constantly destroying our health, life without noticing. How often do you think about healthy eating? Probably only when it becomes really bad, when our body refuses to obey us. We start to use a huge amount of drugs in an attempt to improve our condition. But again we just only poison our body because all drugs contain chemicals which go ill with organs. People! Choose the easier way! Our health comes from the food we eat! Get rid of bad, processed foods, eat healthy and organic, fill your body with vitamins and the result will not keep waiting so long. Your body will begin to rid of toxins and harmful substances in a natural way. You will feel better, your skin, nails and hair will shine with health!

One of the best cleansing (detox) diets is Green Smoothie Cleanse!

What is Green Smoothie Cleanse? Why Green Smoothie? Why 10-Days? What are we eating on this diet? What is the eating plan? Here are the most frequently asked questions. Let's discuss everything like it is.

Judging from the title, we understand that Green Smoothie Detox is based on using green leafy vegetables, fruits and, of course, water. A smoothie is a thick blended beverage, that has "soft, smooth, creamy" texture. Such texture is obtained by whisking the ingredients in a blender. Its consistency, "thickness", depends on the amount of liquid and solid ingredients. Sometimes it is necessary to add different powders (such as protein powder) to thicken your smoothie and make it high-protein. The temperature depends on the temperature of used ingredients: either you use frozen fruits or ice. Smoothie is very nutritious and perfect meal replacement, or energizing, quick and fresh snack

Green Smoothie get their "dark green" "unpleasant" colour from chlorophyll. All leafy veggies such kale, spinach, celery, lettuce contain this nutrient-rich pigment that improves liver function, blood circulation and energize.

## *Why 10-Days?*

Because detoxing process lasts 10 days. You need a period of 10 days, exactly 10 days, to cleanse your body, blood of harmful toxic substances with natural way. It is like a break at school, but "break" for your body, when you detox of highly processed foods, dairy products, meat, and, of course, caffeine. It's not easy! Most of the worst things in life are for free. It is a challenge! You should make efforts and have to be patient and after the first three days you will feel the flow of energy, you'll sleep better, have less bloating and the process of digestion will be improved and the most pleasant thing is – your extra pounds will melt away! This short period helps you to choose the right, healthy way and change your lifestyle.

## 10-Day Green Smoothie Cleanse basic details

<u>Full cleanse</u> – complete cleansing of the body for 10 days. Over a period, you eat three green smoothies, have snacks (celery, carrot, cucumber, apple, peanut butter, only a handful of raw or unsalted nuts, seeds, hard-boiled eggs etc.) and drink filtered water/green tea (8 glasses per day).

<u>Modified cleanse</u> – for those who just want to detox his body, not to lose extra weight. For 10 days you eat two green smoothies for breakfast and lunch, one right healthy meal for dinner (green salad, sautéed vegetables, grilled or baked fish or chicken), have snacks (celery, carrot, cucumber etc.) and drink filtered water/green tea (8 glasses per day).

<u>Breaking the cleanse</u> – it is a period after cleanse. Continue to drink green smoothies twice a day, add salads or sautéed veggies, lean fish and meat for lunch and dinner. Don't go back to unhealthy diet!

<u>Repetition or extension of cleanse</u> – for those who wants to continue lose extra kilos after 20-Days break. Include more protein to your everyday meal. Drink two green smoothies per day, have one healthy, high-protein meal. Have 4-5 meals per day. Drink clean water and green tea.

<u>Continuing to lose weight</u> - lifetime diet – continue to eat unprocessed foods, only healthy fats, low sugar and salt.

The basic requirements for preparing green smoothies

1) All green ingredients for smoothie must be raw.
2) Drink as much water as it possible (about 8 glasses per day).
3) Drink detox and herbal tea (often) (chamomile tea, green tea, peppermint tea, ginger tea, dandelion root tea, milk thistle tea, ginseng tea, sarsaparilla tea)
4) Use only clean, spring or filtered water for your smoothie.
5) Use only organic, ripe, fresh or frozen fruits.
6) Use different ground seeds.
7) Use sweetener if necessary.
8) Use crushed ice or ice cubes.

FOODS TO EAT (Full cleanse and Modified cleanse)

Here the list of recommended greens for your smoothies.

Parsley, carrot top leaves, kale, lettuce, collard greens, dill, turnip greens, spinach, sorrel, mustard greens, bok choy, beet greens, arugula, dandelion greens, watercress.

Green Smoothie = 40% greens + water

Green Smoothie = 40% greens + water + 1 scoop of additional protein powder (rice, hemp, soy protein – NOT whey protein)

Green Smoothie = 40% greens + water + fruits (seedless grapes, mango, blueberries, peaches, bananas, apples, strawberries, pineapples)

Green Smoothie = 40% greens + water + low sugar fruits (lemons, cherries, grapefruits, limes, apples, strawberries, goji berries, blueberries, cranberries)

Green Smoothie = 40% greens + water + moderate sugar fruits (pomegranates, plumps, peaches, oranges, apples, pears)

Green Smoothie = 40% greens + water + high-sugar fruits (apricots, mangos, melons, papayas, kiwis, pineapples, figs, bananas, dates, grapes, raisins).

Typical Detoxification Symptoms

1) You are very hungry and irritable.

2) You have a headache, muscle aches, nausea, fatigue, cravings, skin rashes.

Don't be afraid! You are on the right way! Detoxification starts!

## *FOODS TO AVOID*

(Full cleanse and Modified cleanse)

1) Starchy vegetables (sweet potatoes, beets, carrots, all not leafy greens)

2) Refined and processed foods

3) Refined sugar

4) Refined carbs – pastas, white bread, donuts, etc.

5) Meat

6) Dairy and dairy products – cheese, milk, etc.

7) Dehydrated beverages – (beer, liquor)

8) Coffee and caffeinated beverages

9) Sodas, Cola, diet sodas

10) Fried foods

## *FOODS TO EAT*

(Repetition or extension of cleanse)
1)Dark green leafy/colorful veggies, organic veggies - broccoli, asparagus, cabbage, carrots, garlic, Brussels sprouts, avocados, kale, green beans, spinach, tomatoes, radishes, cucumbers, celery, zucchini, mushrooms etc
2) Flaxseeds, coconut oil, spirulina, bee pollen
3) Clean water, green tea
4) Poultry – skinless chicken, turkey, hen
5) Seafood - clams, lobster, scallops, calamari, crabmeat
6) Fish – wild salmon, sardines, shrimp, trout, tuna, cod, bass, flounder
7) Fruits – all fruits (low-sugar fruits for diabetics)
8) Grains - quinoa, wild rice, bulgur, barley, brown rice, coconut flour, oats
9) Dairy – almond/coconut milk, oat milk, goats milk, eggs, non-dairy butter, plain yogurt
10) Nuts and seeds – hazelnuts, pumpkin seeds, chia seeds, walnuts, peanuts, macadamia nuts, cashews, raw unsalted nuts, almonds, flaxseeds, hemp seeds, sesame seeds etc.
11) Oils – avocado/coconut oil, fish oil, sesame oil, extra-virgin olive oil
12) Sweeteners – raw honey, coconut palm sugar, stevia, monk fruit.
13) Spices – cardamom, black pepper, apple cider, chili peppers, rosemary, sage, saffron, thyme, turmeric, ginger, parsley, dill, cilantro, cinnamon, onion, oregano etc.
14) Beverages – Filtered or spring water, coconut water, fresh juices, green/black/mint tea, herbal tea

FOODS TO AVOID (Repetition or extension of cleanse)
1) Processed and fatty meat – hot dogs, salami, sausage, bacon, prime rib, porterhouse
2) Vegetables – red/white potato
3) Fruits – canned/dried fruits
4) Grains – bread, pasta, rice
5) Sugar, salt, coffee, fruit juice, ketchup, mayonnaise,
6) Dairy – cheese, cream cheese, sour cream, powdered milk, fruit yogurt.
7) Oils – trans fats, vegetable oils, margarine, bacon/chicken fat
8) Beverages – sodas, Cola, fruit juice, beer

## *Why Greens?*

The Best Greens For Your Green Smoothie Recipes

**Arugula** – contains vitamins C, K, A, minerals, antioxidants, high levels of folic acid, potassium, manganese, iron, calcium. Arugula is rich on phytochemicals, which prevents cancer.

**Broccoli** - contains vitamin B (except B12), copper, phosphorus, potassium. It is rich in antioxidants which help to reduce the risk of cervical, breast and prostate cancer and boosts liver function.

**Collard**  - is a source of vitamin B. Also it contains vitamins A, C, K, manganese, calcium. It is an excellent antioxidant. Collard greens has an ability to support natural detoxification, it has anti-inflammatory effect, prevents cancer and supports cardiovascular system.

**Cilantro** - contains vitamins A, C, E, K, iron, calcium, potassium, magnesium. Cilantro is an anti-diabetic plant. Calcium content strengthens bones, hair, nails and teeth. Constant usage of cilantro supports cardiovascular system, lowers cholesterol and blood pressure.

**Chickweed** - contains calcium, magnesium, iron, manganese, silica, sodium, selenium, phosphorus, zinc and potassium. It is rich in vitamins A, B-1, B-2, C. It has laxative effect and helps to detox body.  with natural way. Chickweed is a natural antiseptic and often used for wound healing.

**Chicory** – improves digestion processes, prevents heartburn, lowers arthritis pains and inflammatory processes. Chicory prevents bacterial infections, improves your immune system. It has sedative effect and fights toxins, it helps to detoxify liver. Using chicory in your smoothies promotes extra weight loss.

**Dandelion Greens** – contain vitamins C, B, E, iron, potassium, zinc, copper, phosphorous, magnesium, calcium. Improves the production of bile that, in turn, improves liver function. Strengthen the immune system and helps to fight cancer cells.

**Dill** – is one of the best sources of calcium, iron, manganese and vitamin C. Dill is an antioxidant food, that's why it has an anti-inflammatory effect. It lowers the level of cholesterol, treats epilepsy symptoms.  As dill is rich in vitamin C it boosts our body with energy, improves immunity system, aids in digestion.

**Fennel**  - contains vitamin C, potassium, iron, manganese, folate, fiber. It is enriched with phytonutrients and volatile oils. Fennel settles digestion and help fight extra pounds. This green superfood has a diuretic effect and improves kidneys work.

**Grape Leaves** -  are low-calorie greens (about 14 calories per every 5 leaves) and powerful antioxidant. Grape leaves are a good source of vitamins C, E, A, K, B6, niacin, fiber, iron, riboflavin, calcium, folate, magnesium, manganese and copper. Grape leaves are fat and cholesterol-free. And has low sodium and sugar content. That's why it helps to control blood glucose level. Vitamin C promotes good digestion and strengthens immune system.

**Lettuce** - is an "excellent weight loss food", that rich in vitamins and minerals. It helps to detox body and improves digestion. It is very nutritious and low sugar superfood.

**Kale** –  is the king of greens and weight loss friendly food. It contains protein, calcium, vitamin K, iron, vitamin C, A, magnesium etc. It is a powerful antioxidant. Thanks to variety of vitamins and minerals, kale lowers cholesterol, reduces the risk of heart diseases, protects from cancer.

**Microgreens** – is a powerful antioxidant and very nutritious ingredient. These small greens are enriched with vitamins C, E, K and have a high level of beta-carotene that prevents you from eye diseases and type II diabetes.

**Mint** – this green herb is one of the most powerful antioxidants. And as it known, antioxidants play an important role in preventing people's health from cancer, heart disease and Alzheimer's. it improves liver function and relieve asthma symptoms. Mint is a great relaxant, it is usually used in cocktails and different kinds of tea. Due to the variety of enzymes mint is found as a strong cancer-fighting agent.

**Mustard** - contains vitamins A, K, carotenes, iron, calcium, magnesium, zinc, potassium, selenium, and manganese. It is a weight loss friendly food because leaf-mustard is low in calories. It also helps to control cholesterol level and prevents arthritis, iron deficiency anemia, osteoporosis and protects from cardiovascular diseases, prostate cancers and asthma.

**Parsley** – one of the most widespread green smoothie ingredient. This fragrant herb is rich in vitamins A, K, C, E, B6, B12, thiamin, niacin, riboflavin, pantothenic acid, folates, choline, calcium, magnesium, iron, manganese, potassium, phosphorous, zinc and copper. It has anti-diabetic properties because decreases blood sugar levels. Thanks to vitamin C and beta-carotene, parsley has an anti-inflammatory properties. It controls kidney stones, gallbladder stones and urinary tract infections thanks to its diuretic effect.

 **Purslane** – has high levels of omega-3 fatty acids, great amounts of fiber and is rich in vitamins A, C, B, iron, manganese, potassium, magnesium, calcium and copper. It helps to cleanse the body and aids to fight obesity. Thanks to its properties, purslane improves heart functioning, possesses healthy growth and development of children, prevents cancer and strengthen the immune system.

**Spinach** -  is rich in vitamins C, E, K, A, B2, B6, manganese, magnesium, Iron, calcium, potassium. Spinach is an excellent source of antioxidants, that's why it has an excellent anti-inflammatory effect. It has anti-cancer fighting agents and boosts immunity.

**Watercress** – provides great nutrition, strengthen immunity, prevents cancer. It is enriched with vitamins C, A, B6, B12 calcium, iron, magnesium, folate, phosphorus which are all required for a healthy body. It helps to prevent breast cancer, improves thyroid gland functioning, cardiovascular health and bone health.

*Variety of Green Smoothie for your health*

For Slimming -  the best combination is greens + fruits +chia seeds.  This unbelievable combination provides the feeling of satiety. Chia seeds combined with leafy greens and fruits help you to forget about eating for many hours. Chia seeds and aloe vera are natural purgatives that promote good digestion and help your body to get rid of toxins.

For Getting the Boost of Energy -  just add super energizing ingredients as goji, pine pollen, astragalus or ginseng extracts, moringa, spirulina to your green smoothie and feel unbelievable energy inflow.

For people with diabetes – the main requirement for green smoothie is a low sugar content or its  total absence. We usually use frozen ingredients such bananas, mangos for thickness and sweetness of our smoothie. But neither in this case! We need other ingredients that help to control blood sugar levels. The excellent variant is chia seeds. This ingredient makes your smoothie thicker and generates "sweet taste". Also combine green apples, goji, kiwi, blueberries, magui berries, acai powder, stevia extract and be sure that your green smoothie is a safe choice!

For Gaining a Muscle Bulk -  if you are striving to gain muscle bulk -  drink high-protein dark green smoothies! Use natural protein-rich foods like kale, collard. Combine them with raw protein powders, hemp protein, add fats - coconut kefir, maca, spirulina, crushed nuts, seeds pine pollen and be sure that it is really natural, right and high-protein smoothie!

For Little Gourmets -  the color of green smoothie is not popular with children! But be smarter! Firstly, limit the volume of green ingredients. Use more sweet, colourful fruits with nut milk.  But when the little gourmets can't live without his beloved smoothies, start adding more greens. Smoothies will be more nutritious!

## RECIPES

### *1. Spinach, Green Apple, and Kiwi Green Smoothie*

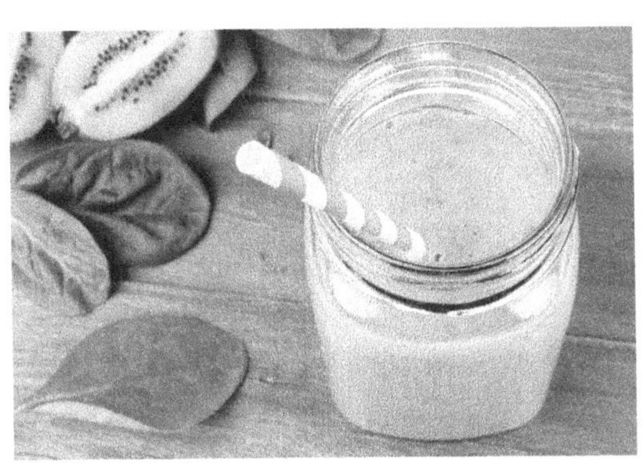

<u>**INGREDIENTS**</u> for 4 servings
Chia seeds – 10 gr
Water – 120 ml
Apple juice – 150ml
Green apples – 1 piece
Kiwi – 1 piece
Fresh mint – 5 pcs
Iswari chlorella – 1 tsp
Spinach leaves – ¼ cup

## <u>INSTRUCTIONS</u>
1. Firstly, soak chia seeds in water for 1-2 min.
2. Meanwhile, dice apple and kiwi, chop spinach leaves. Put all ingredients and soaked seeds in blender.
3. Blend until creamy.
<u>Nutritional values (for 1 serving)</u>
Carbs - 14 g, fiber - 2 g, protein - 1 g, fat – 0,5 g, energy – 60 kcal

## *2. Spinach, Blueberry, Strawberry, Apple, Orange, Banana Green Smoothie*

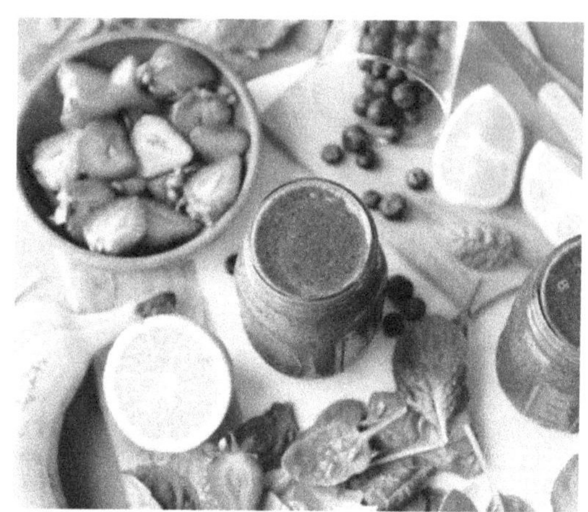

## **INGREDIENTS**
Apple -  1 piece
Banana – 1 piece
Blueberries – 150 gr
Oranges – 1 piece
Spinach – 30 gr
Strawberries – 12 gr
Water – 4240 ml

## **INSTRUCTIONS**
1. Put all ingredients in blender.
2. Blend until smooth.
Nutritional values (for 1/3 of recipe – 473 gr)
Carbs - 40 g, fiber - 7 g, protein - 3 g, fat – 1 g, energy – 156 kcal

### *3. Low Sugar Green Smoothie*

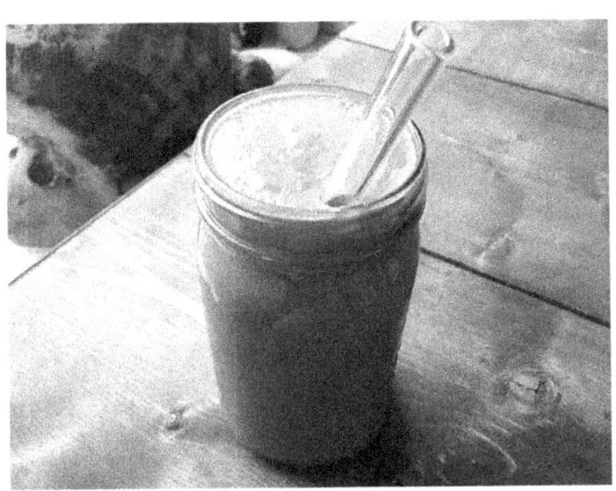

## INGREDIENTS

Water – 240 ml
Avocado – 1 piece
Kale – 30 gr
Spinach – 30 gr
Lemon juice -  15 ml
Ginger – 10 gr

## INSTRUCTIONS

1. Peel and chop avocado, remove stems_from the kale.
2. Put in blender. Blend until smooth.
3. Enjoy!
Nutritional values (per 1 serving)
Carbs - 33 g, protein - 5 g, fat – 29 g, energy – 400 kcal

## *4. Antioxidant Green Smoothie with Pomegranate*

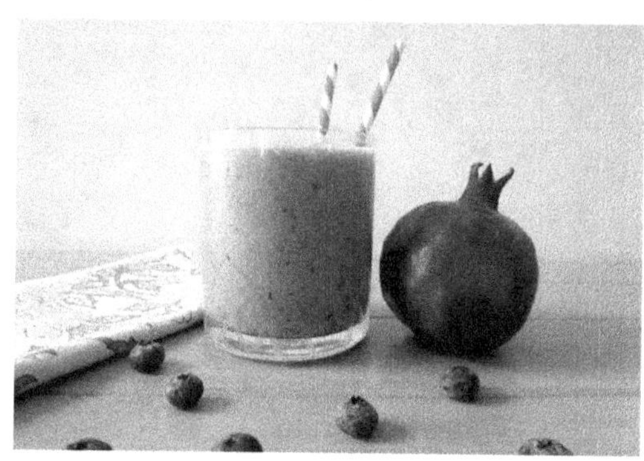

## <u>INGREDIENTS</u>

Pomegranate seeds – ½ cup
Frozen blueberries – 1 cup
Peeled banana – 1 piece   peeled
Frozen raspberries – ½ cup
Cacao powder – 10 gr
Baby spinach – 100 gr
Unsweetened almond milk – 225 gr

## <u>INSTRUCTIONS</u>

1. Firstly, pour almond milk into blender bowl, then add pomegranate seeds, frozen berries, banana and at the end add cacao powder and spinach.
2. Blend until creamy consistency.
3. Drizzle with pomegranate seeds on the top. Enjoy!
<u>Nutritional values (per 1 serving)</u>
Carbs - 78 g, protein - 9 g, fiber - 20.7g fat – 3 g, energy – 375 kcal

## *5. A very refreshing healthy smoothie*

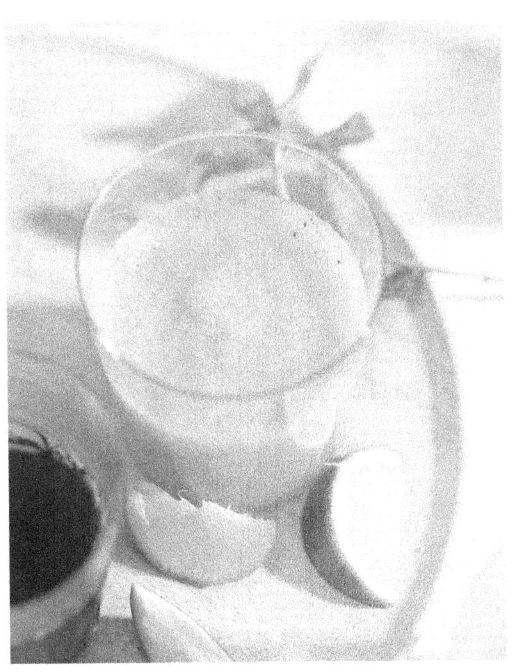

**INGREDIENTS** (for 1 serving)
Caffeine-free green or white tea - 1 bag
Water - 160 ml
Mango – ½ cup
Fresh lime juice – 5 ml
Crushed ice – 2 cups

**INSTRUCTIONS**
1. Make the tea. Cool it. Cut mango into cubes.
2. Put all ingredients in the blender, pour cooled tea and blend until thick and smooth.
3. Add crushed ice.
4. Enjoy immediately!
Nutritional values (per 1 serving)
Carbs – 14,4 g, protein – 0,4 g, fiber – 1,5 g fat – 0,2 g, energy – 54,9 kcal

## *6. Orange, Strawberry, Banana and Spinach Smoothie*

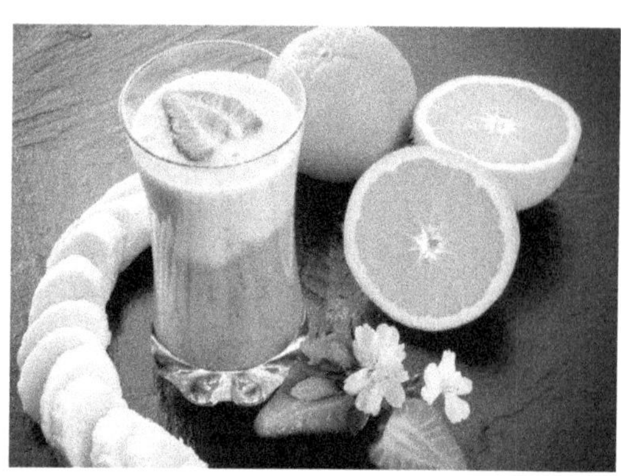

**INGREDIENTS** (for 1 serving )
Spinach leaves – 50 gr
Banana – 1 piece
Strawberries – 7 pcs
Orange juice – 180 ml

**INSTRUCTIONS**
1. Put all ingredients in your bender.
2. Blend until smooth.
3. Drink cool!
Nutritional values (per 1 serving)
Carbs – 55,9 g, protein – 5,2 g, fiber – 6,4 g fat – 1,4 g, energy – 233,9 kcal

## *7. Green Smoothie: Spinach, Banana & Strawberry*

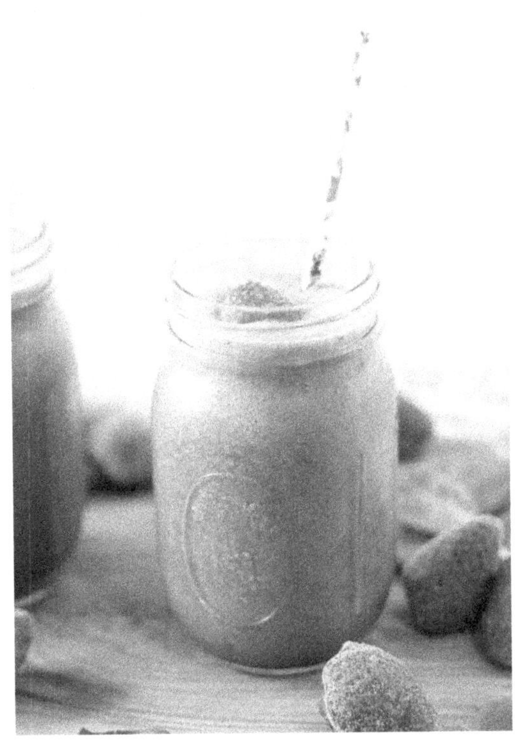

## <u>INGREDIENTS</u> (for 1 serving)

Water – 240 ml
Baby spinach – 85 gr
Banana – 1 piece
Strawberries – 4 pcs

## <u>INSTRUCTIONS</u>
1. Slice banana and strawberries.
2. Place all smoothie ingredients in your blender. Blend until smooth.
3. Enjoy!

<u>Nutritional values (per 1 serving)</u>
Carbs – 38,3 g, protein – 3,6 g, fiber – 6,5 g fat – 1 g, energy – 156,9 kcal

## *8. Green Monster Smoothie*

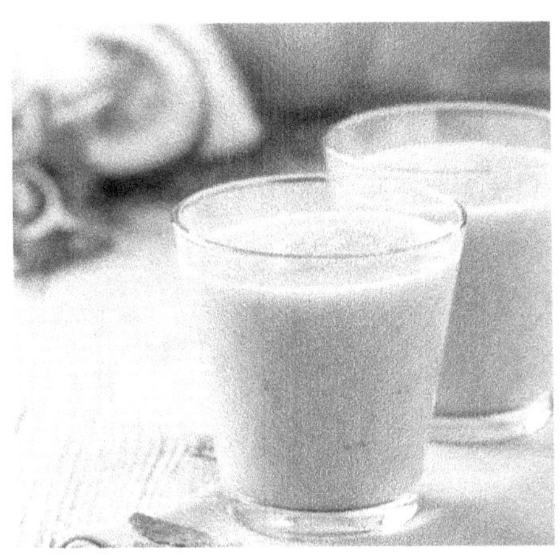

**INGREDIENTS** (for 2 servings)
Peach- 1 piece
Baby spinach – 85 gr
Soy Milk – 120 ml
Water – 240 ml (optional)

**INSTRUCTIONS**
1. Combine peach, milk and water in a blender. At the end add spinach. Blend well.
2. Enjoy!
Nutritional values (per 1 serving)
Carbs – 11,9 g, protein – 2,8 g, fiber – 3,2 g fat – 0,5 g, energy – 56,1 kcal

## *9. Green Smoothie*

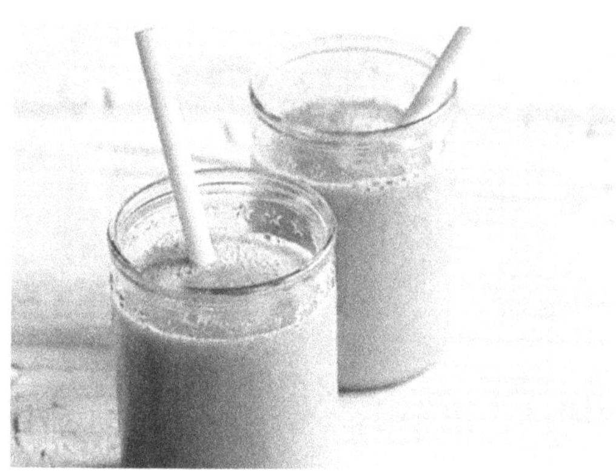

## **INGREDIENTS** (for 2 servings)

Milk – 240 ml
Spinach – 85 gr
Fresh pineapple – 225 gr
Grapes – 200 gr
Ice
Sweetness if you like

## **INSTRUCTIONS**
1. Take a high powered mixer. Combine all smoothie ingredients and blend.
2. Add your favorite sweetness if you desire.

## *10. Collard Green Pineapple Smoothie*

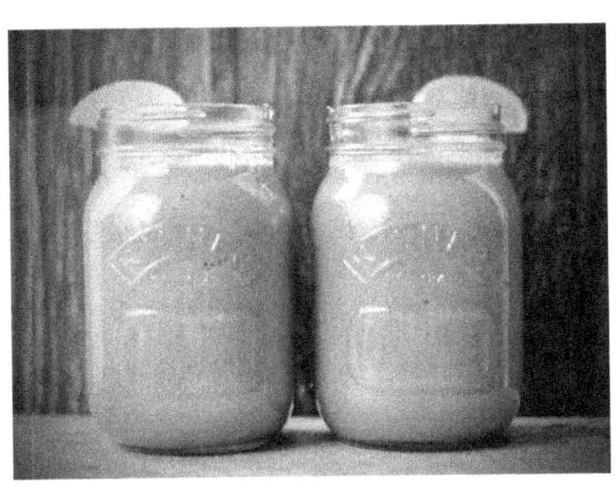

**INGREDIENTS** (for 1 serving)
Banana – 1 piece   or 2 extra small bananas
Collards (chopped) – ½ cup
Pineapple (chopped) – ½ cup
Water – 120 ml

**INSTRUCTIONS**
1. Place all smoothie ingredients in a blender.
2. Pulverize until smooth. Light green collard green pineapple smoothie is ready!
3. Enjoy!
Nutritional values (per 1 serving)
Carbs – 53 g, protein – 3,9 g, fiber – 6,6 g fat – 1,1 g, energy – 215,7 kcal

## *11. Funny Green Smoothie*

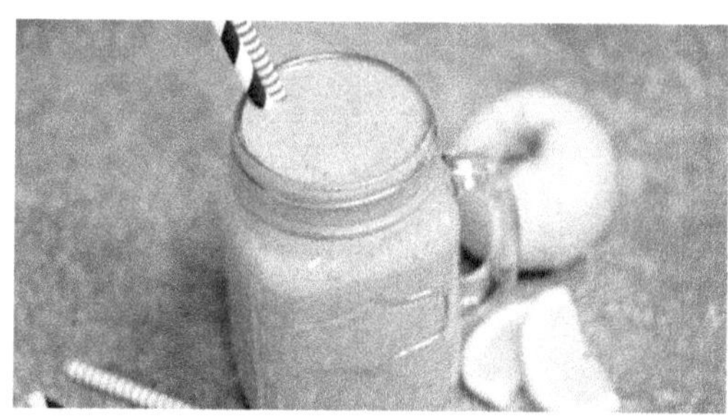

<u>**INGREDIENTS**</u> (for 1 serving)
Frozen banana – 1 piece
Frozen fruit mixture (pineapple, peaches, strawberries) – ¼ cup
Bee pollen – 5gr
Water – 60 ml
Pomegranate juice – 60 ml
Spinach – ½ cup
Kale – ½ cup

## **INSTRUCTIONS**

1. Combine bee pollen and water. Mix.
2. Now put fruits, juice, spinach and kale in a blender. Blend well.
3. Enjoy immediately!
<u>Nutritional values (per 1 serving)</u>
Carbs –44,6 g, protein – 4,3 g, fiber – 4,5 g fat – 1,3 g, energy – 184,2 kcal

## *12. Chocolate Strawberry Green Smoothie*

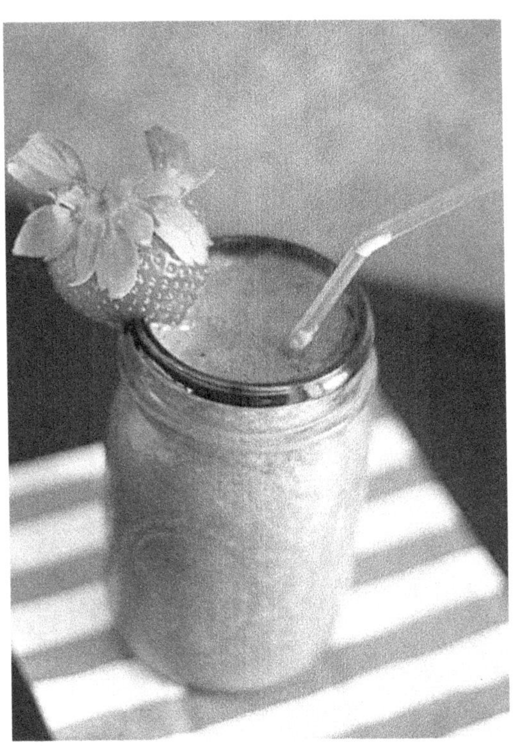

**INGREDIENTS** (for 1 serving)
Chocolate protein powder - 0.75 scoop
Chocolate Amazing Grass - 0.25 scoop (optional)
Low fat goat's milk – 60 ml
Spinach – 30 gr
Frozen strawberries – 1 cup
Water – 120 ml
Ice cubes

**INSTRUCTIONS**
1. Firstly, combine chocolate protein powder, chocolate Amazing Grass and milk. Blend until smooth.

2. Then put chopped spinach, frozen strawberries, pour water. Blend again.
3. Finally, add ice cubes.

<u>Nutritional values (per 1 serving)</u>
Carbs –25,8 g, protein – 25,9 g, fiber – 8,0 g fat – 1,3 g, energy – 207,1 kcal

## *13. Pomegranate-Pluot Green Smoothie*

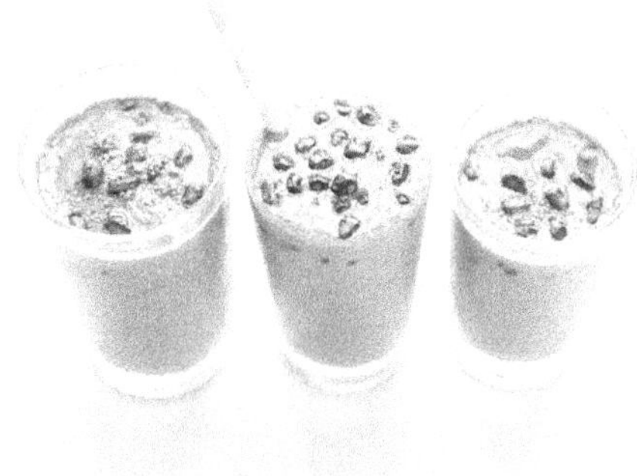

**<u>INGREDIENTS</u>** ( for 1 serving)
Pomegranate seeds – ½ cup
Banana – 1 piece
Plum – 1 piece
Cucumber – ¼
Romaine lettuce – 1 head
Water – 230 ml

## <u>INSTRUCTIONS</u>
1. Peel banana, cut cucumber into pieces and pit the plum.
2. Place these ingredients in a blender. Pulverize until homogeneous consistency.
<u>Nutritional values (per 1 serving)</u>
Carbs –75 g, protein – 8 g, fiber – 8,0 g fat – 2 g, energy – 321 kcal

## *14. Sugar-free Green Smoothie*

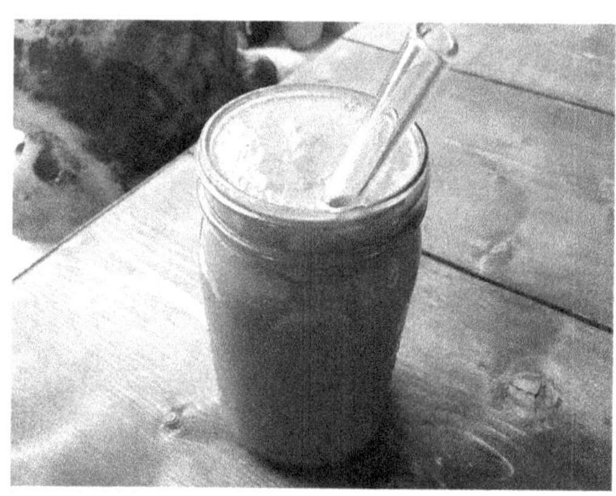

**INGREDIENTS** (for 2 servings)
Half of one avocado
Apples – 4 pcs
Lime – 1/4
Cucumber- 1/4
Celery stalk – 1 piece
Spinach – 1 handful

## **INSTRUCTIONS**
1. Peel 1 apple, avocado and lime. Put all ingredients except for one apple and half of one avocado in a juicer.
2. Then put peeled and chopped apple and scoop out avocado. Put them in a blender.
3. Pour in juice and add Ice. Blend until smooth.
Nutritional values (per 1 serving)
Carbs –82,9 g, protein – 3,2 g, fiber – 13,6 g fat – 8,1 g, energy – 380,2 kcal

## *15. Green Monster Smoothie*

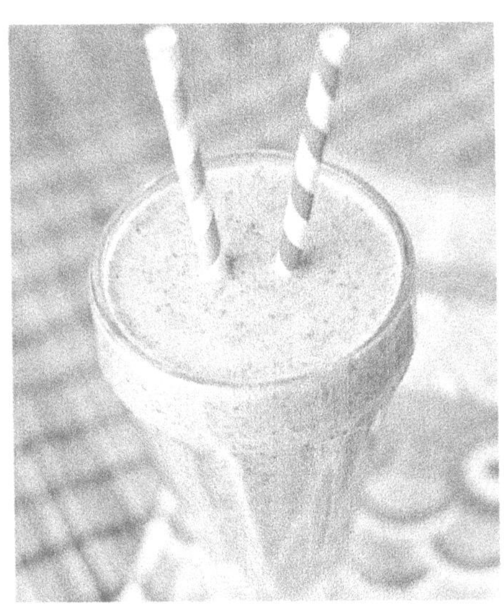

## **INGREDIENTS** (for 1 serving)
Skim milk – 240ml
Banana – 1 piece
Ground flax – 30 gr
Almond butter – 15 gr
Fresh baby spinach – 70 gr
Ice cubes – 5 pcs

## **INSTRUCTIONS**
1. Combine and blend all ingredients.
2. Enjoy!
Nutritional values (per 1 serving)
Carbs –49,3 g, protein – 17,3 g, fiber – 8,7 g fat – 14,8 g, energy – 373,6 kcal

## *16. Creamy Green Smoothie*

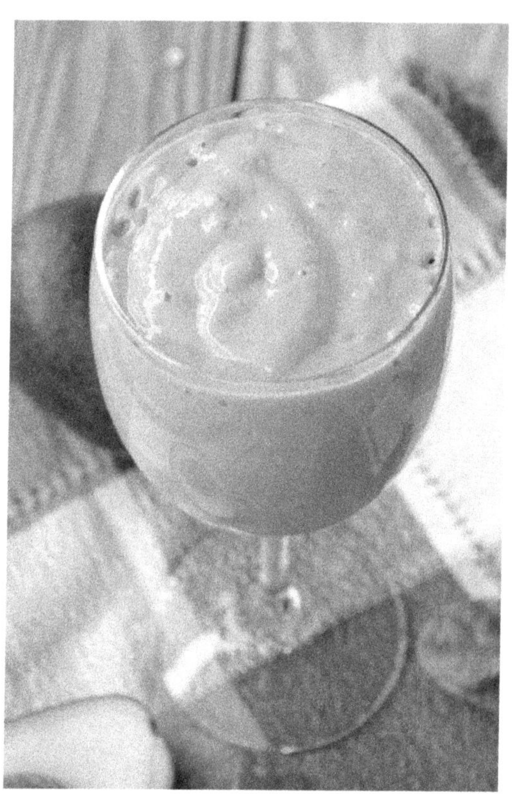

**<u>INGREDIENTS</u>** (for 1 serving)
Water – 230 ml
Baby spinach – 1 handful
Half of one avocado
Half of one banana
Half of one lime
Ice – 1 handful

**<u>INTRUCTIONS</u>**
1. Combine and blend all ingredients.
2. Add ice and blend once again.

3. Squeeze with lime juice. Enjoy!

<u>Nutritional values (per 1 serving)</u>
Carbs –25,4 g, protein – 2,7 g, fiber – 9,1 g fat – 13,7 g, energy – 212,2 kcal

## *17. Collard Green Mango Smoothie*

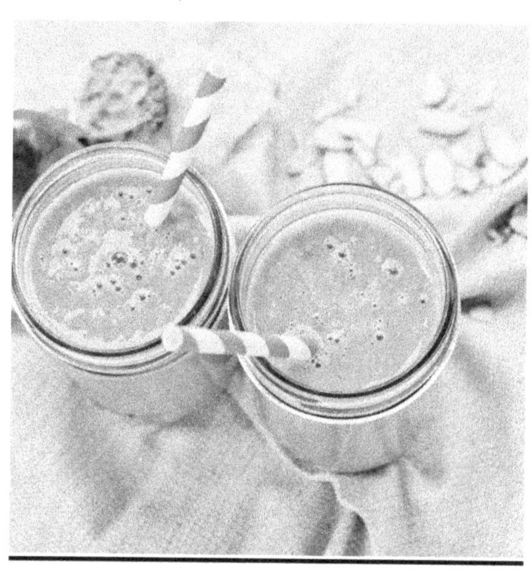

**<u>INGREDIENTS</u>** (for 1 serving)
Frozen mangoes (chopped) – 1 cup
Fresh banana – 1 piece
Water – 115 ml
Collard greens (chopped0 – 1 cup

**<u>INTRUCTIONS</u>**
1. Chop mangoes and collard greens.
2. Put in a blender and pulverize.
3. Pour in two glasses.
<u>Nutritional values (per 1 serving)</u>
Carbs – 60,8 g, protein – 4 g, fiber – 8,8 g fat – 1,1 g, energy – 240,8 kcal

## *18. Green Monster Smoothie (for energy, hair, nail strength and clear skin)*

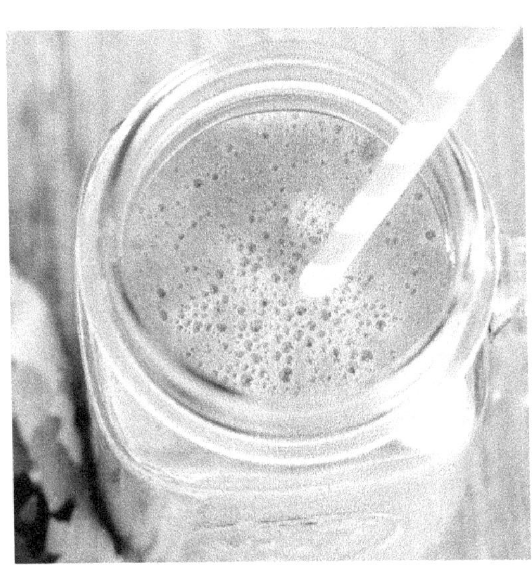

**INGREDIENTS** (for 1 serving)
Baby spinach - 1,5cup
Frozen pineapple – 1 cup
Banana – 1 piece
Flax seed – 15 gr
Almond milk – 240 ml

**INTRUCTIONS**
1. Combine all ingredients in a blender bowl. Mix until smooth.
2. Add crushed ice if you like thick smoothie.
Nutritional values (per 1 serving)
Carbs – 49,4 g, protein – 5,2 g, fiber – 8,5 g fat – 7 g, energy – 264,5 kcal

## *19. Super Size Green Smoothie*

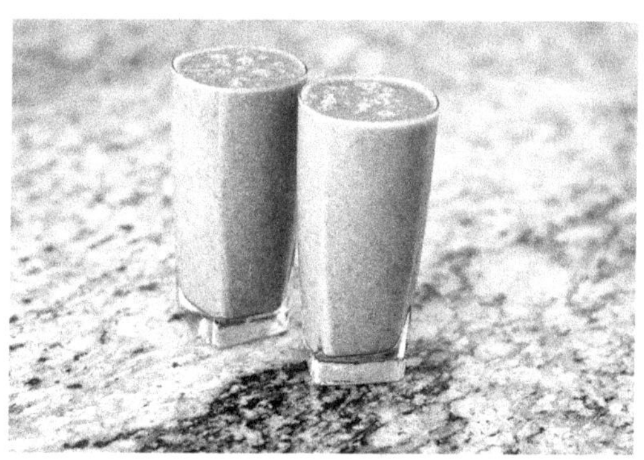

## <u>**INGREDIENTS**</u> (for 1 serving)
Aloe Vera Gel – 115 gr
Organic Kefir – 56 gr
Frozen cranberries – 7 gr
Raspberries – 14 gr
Watermelon – 1 slice
Protein Powder - Nutribiotic Rice – 30 gr
Protein Powder - Nature's Way Alive Ultra Shake – 30 gr
Protein Powder - Nutiva Hemp – 15 gr
Bee Pollen – 15 gr
Vitamineral Green Powder – 15 gr
Chlorella – 7 gr
Fresh Swiss Chard – 1 cup
Kale – 1 cup
Spinach – 1 cup
Orange – 1 piece
Apple – 1 piece
Pear – 1 piece
Kiwi – 1 piece
Grapes – 20 pcs

Pineapple – 1 slice
Banana – 1 piece

## **INTRUCTIONS**
1. Put liquid ingredients and watermelon slice in a blender. Blend.
2. Add fresh Swiss chard, kale, spinach. Blend again.
3. Add fruits. Blend until smooth.
4. Divide into several portions.
Nutritional values (per 1 serving)
Carbs – 207,2 g, protein – 40,2 g, fiber – 30,3 g fat – 7 g, energy – 974 kcal

## *20. Green Smoothie*

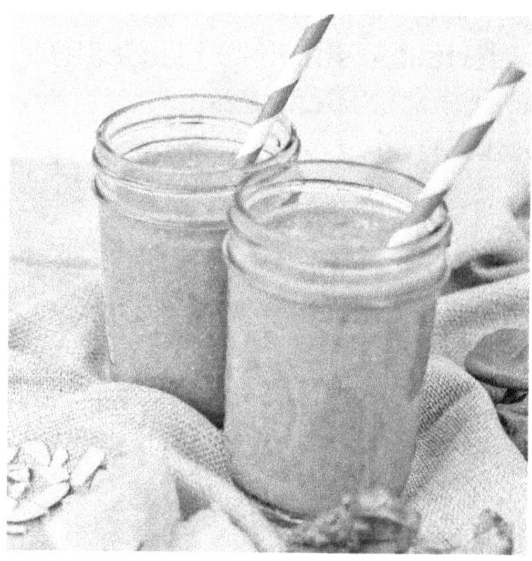

**<u>INGREDIENTS</u>** <u>(for 4 serving)</u>
Tomatoes – 2 pcs
Carrots – 2 pcs
Celery – 2 stalks
Spinach – 2 cups
Half of one green bell pepper
Bell Pepper – ¼ cup
Worcestershire sauce – 15 ml
Broccoli
Hot sauce, salt to taste

## <u>INTRUCTIONS</u>
1. Use high-speed and powerful blender. Combine all smoothie ingredients and blend for 1 minute.
<u>Nutritional values (per 1 serving)</u>
Carbs – 5,5 g, protein – 1,2 g, fiber – 1,6 g fat – 0,2 g, energy – 25,3 kcal

## *21. Kale Green Smoothie*

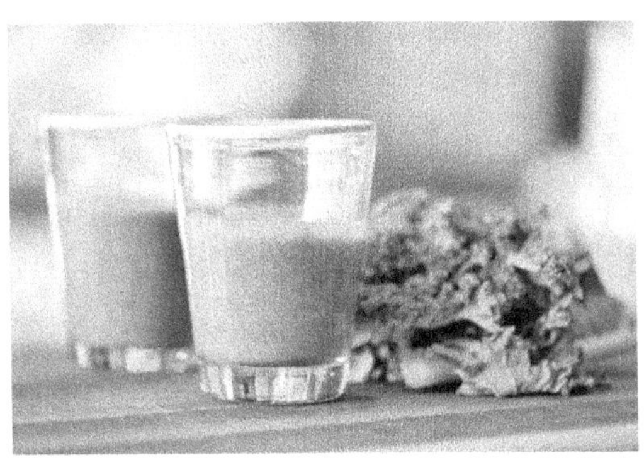

## INGREDIENTS (for 2 serving)
Water – 120-240 ml
Fresh kale – 2 cups
Mango – 1 piece
Banana – 1 piece
Ground flaxseed – 30 gr

## INSTRUCTIONS
1. Make preparations: peel and pit mango. Cut into chunks.  Ground flaxseeds.
2. Pour water in blender and add fresh kale. Blend.
3. Put in mango chunks, peeled banana slices and ground flaxseed.
4. Blend until smooth. If desired, dilute with water.
5. Enjoy with ice or chilled!
NOTE You may keep this amazing Kale Green Smoothie in your fridge for two days.
Nutritional values (per 1 serving)
Carbs – 42,1 g, protein – 5,6 g, fiber – 8,4 g fat – 5,1 g, energy – 212,9 kcal

## *22. Refreshing Green Smoothie*

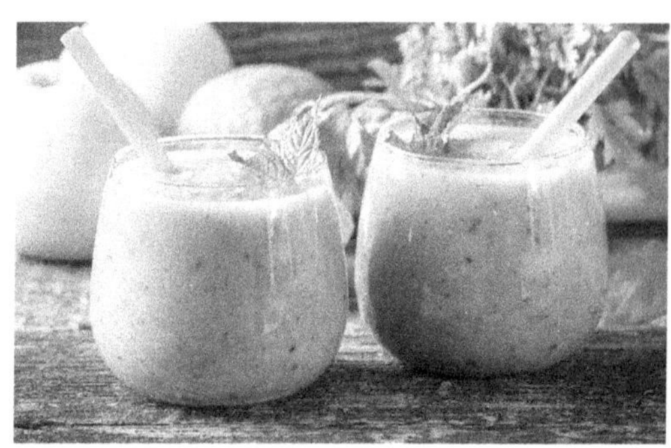

**INGREDIENTS** (for 1 serving)
Fresh spinach – 30 gr
Cucumber – ¼ cup
Half of one fresh banana
Fresh pineapple – ½ cup
Vanilla yogurt – 100 ml
Juice – 120 ml (any you like)

**INSTRUCTIONS**
1. Mix all smoothie ingredients in a blender. Pulse.
2. If desired, add ice and pulse once again.
Nutritional values (per 1 serving)
Carbs – 55 g, protein – 7,6 g, fiber – 3,7 g fat – 2,7 g, energy – 260,7 kcal

## *23. Green POWER Smoothie*

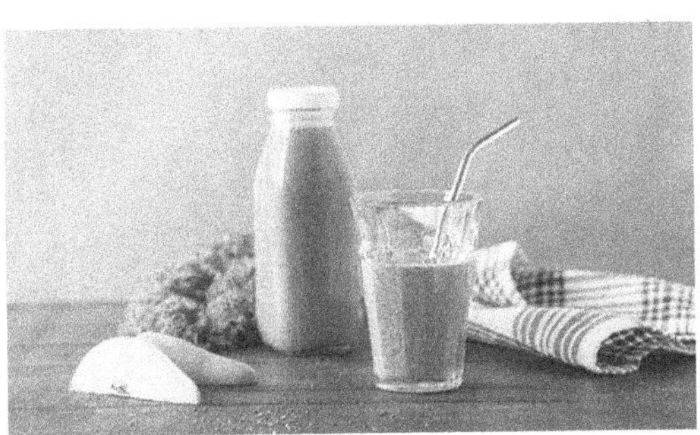

**INGREDIENTS** (for 1 serving)

Frozen banana – 1 piece
Frozen pineapple – 1 cup
Spinach – 1 handful
Coconut water – 240 ml
Vanilla whey protein – 1 scoop

**INSTRUCTIONS**
1. To prepare this Power smoothie, use high-speed blender.
2. Combine all ingredients in a blender bowl. Pulse until smooth.
3. Taste it!
Nutritional values (per 1 serving)
Carbs – 52,2 g, protein – 27 g, fiber – 4,4 g fat – 2,2 g, energy – 316 kcal

## *24. St. Patrick's Day Green Smoothie*

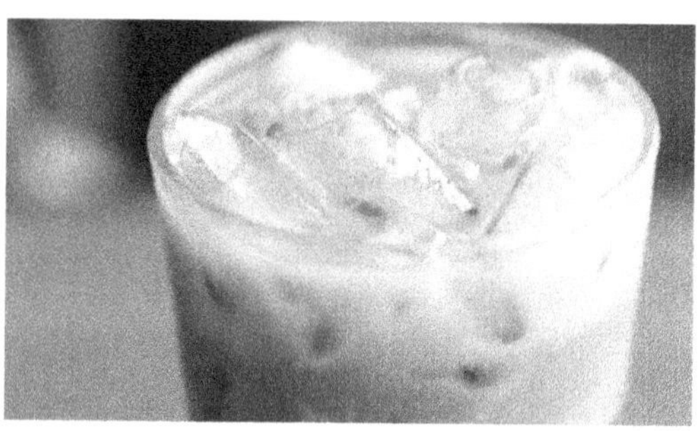

**INGREDIENTS** (for 1 serving)
Fruit mixture – 1 cup (peaches, strawberries, red grapes, honey dew melon, pineapple)
Vanilla Rice Dream – 1 cup
Kale – 30 gr
Banana – 1 piece
Water – 120 ml

**INSTRUCTIONS**
1. Place all of the ingredients in a blender. Pulse until smooth.
2. Enjoy!
Nutritional values (per 1 serving)
Carbs – 77 g, protein – 5,8 g, fiber – 10,3 g fat – 3,6 g, energy – 339,3 kcal

## 25. *Green Monster Smoothie*

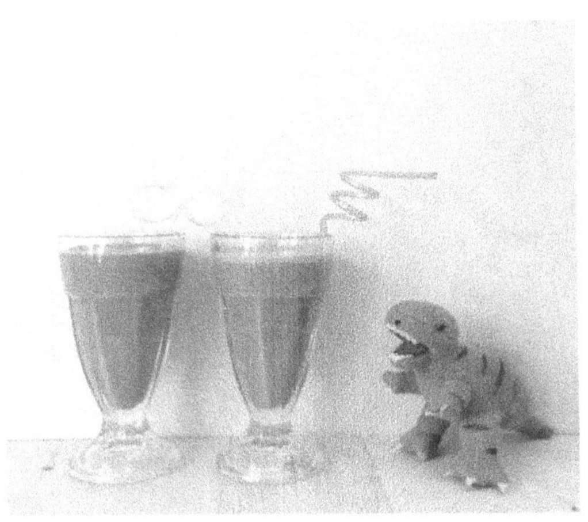

## <u>INGREDIENTS</u> (for 2 serving)

Raw baby spinach – 70 gr
Soy or almond milk – 240 ml
Water – 120 ml
Plain yogurt – 2-3 tsp
Granny Smith apple – 1 piece (unpeeled)
Banana – 1piece
Stevia – 1 packet

## <u>INSTRUCTIONS</u>
1. Firstly, blend raw baby spinach, milk, water, plain yogurt.
2. Then add cored apple and peeled banana. Blend again.
3. At the end add 1 stevia packet.  Blend until fluffy and smooth.
4. Pour into glasses.
<u>Nutritional values (per 1 serving)</u>
Carbs – 33.1 g, protein – 6,7 g, fiber – 3,9 g fat – 1,2 g, energy – 156,2 kcal

## *26. Extra Virgin Coconut Oil and Oats Green Smoothie*

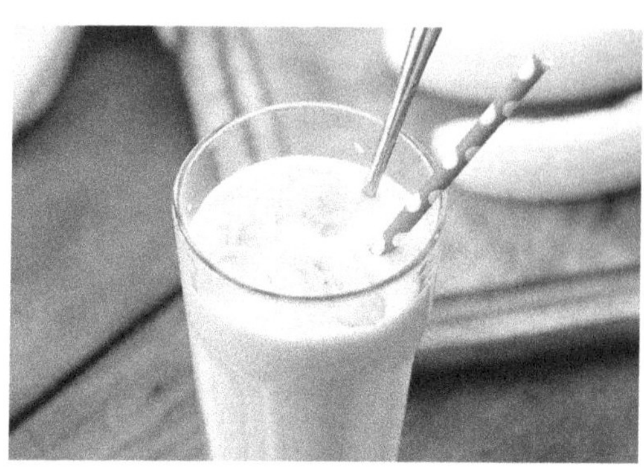

**INGREDIENTS** (for 1 serving)
Fat free milk – 240 ml
Water – 240 ml
Carnantion vanilla instant breakfast – 0,5 packet
Frozen pineapple chucks – 1 cup
Kale – 1 bunch
Uncooked old fashion oats – ½ cup
Extra Virgin Coconut Oil – 15 gr

**INSTRUCTIONS**
1. Melt oil.
2. Combine all smoothie ingredients. Blend and drink immediately!
Nutritional values (per 1 serving)
Carbs – 78,9 g, protein – 19 g, fiber – 8,5 g fat – 18,2 g, energy – 530,4 kcal

## *27. My Favorite Green Smoothie!*

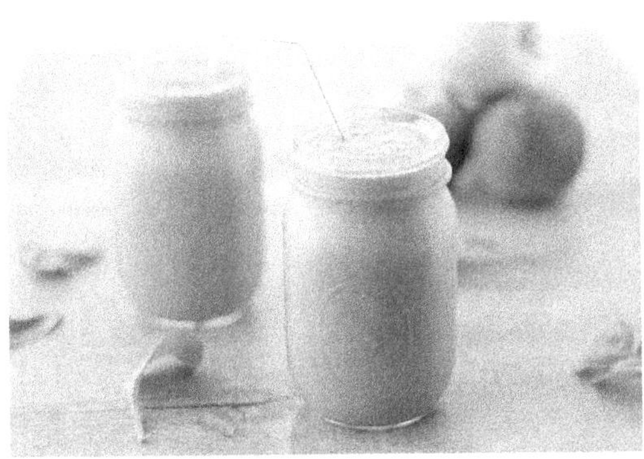

**<u>INGREDIENTS</u>** <u>(for 2 serving)</u>
Fresh spinach – 4 cups
Water - 480 ml
Frozen banana – 3 pcs
Fresh apples – 1 piece
Fresh pear – 1 piece
Fresh grapes – 1 cup

**<u>INSTRUCTIONS</u>**
1. Remove seeds from the apple, grapes and pear.
2. Pour water in a blender and add fresh spinach. Blend well.
3. Then add peeled bananas. Pulse.
4. Then apple, pear chunks and grapes. Pulse well.
5. Add ice cubes and enjoy!
<u>Nutritional values (per 1 serving)</u>
Carbs – 70,5 g, protein – 4,1 g, fiber – 8,8 g fat – 2 g, energy – 255,4 kcal

## *28. Winter Green Smoothie*

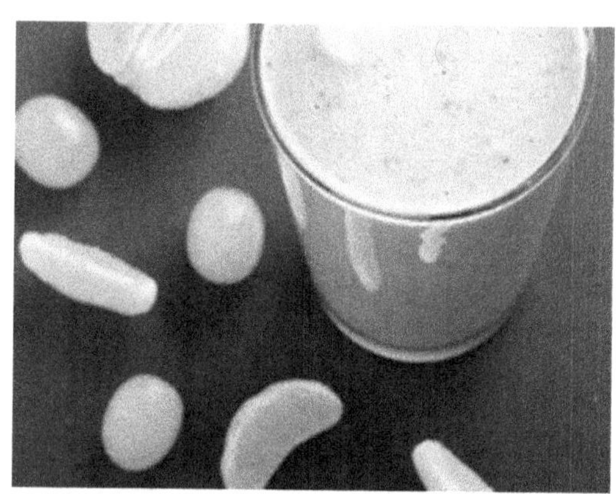

**<u>INGREDIENTS</u>** (for 2 serving)
Apples – 2 pcs
Pears – 2 pcs
Frozen cranberries – one handful
Water – 480 ml
Kale leaves – 7 pcs
Collard greens – 5 pcs
Green cabbage – 1 chunk
Fresh ginger
Fresh parsley

## <u>INSTRUCTIONS</u>
1. Core apples and pears, cut into chunks.
2. Combine ingredients except greens. Blend.
3. Throw greens and blend again until smooth.
4. If desired, dissolve thick smoothie with water.
NOTE Keep in fridge for one day.
<u>Nutritional values (per 1 serving)</u>
Carbs – 62, 7 g, protein – 4, 1 g, fiber – 14, 3 g, fat – 1, 8 g, energy – 252, 3 kcal

## *29. CREAMY GINGER GREEN SMOOTHIE*

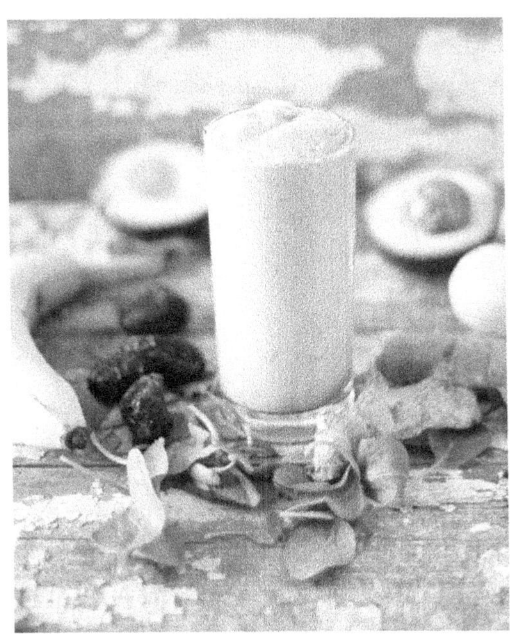

**INGREDIENTS** (for 1 serving)
Organic spinach – 2 handfuls
Water – 240 ml
Half of one avocado
Banana – 1 piece
Tahini – 1 tbsp
Dates – 2 pcs (pitted)
Fresh chopped ginger root – to taste
Meyer lemon juice

**INSTRUCTIONS**
1. Just put all ingredients into a blender and pulse until creamy and thick.
2. Add ice if you like cool smoothie.
3. Enjoy!

<u>Nutritional values (per 1 serving)</u>
Carbs – 49 g, protein – 5 g, fiber – 11 g, fat – 21 g, energy – 390 kcal, sugar - 15

## *30. Pineapple-Broccoli Green Smoothie Recipe*

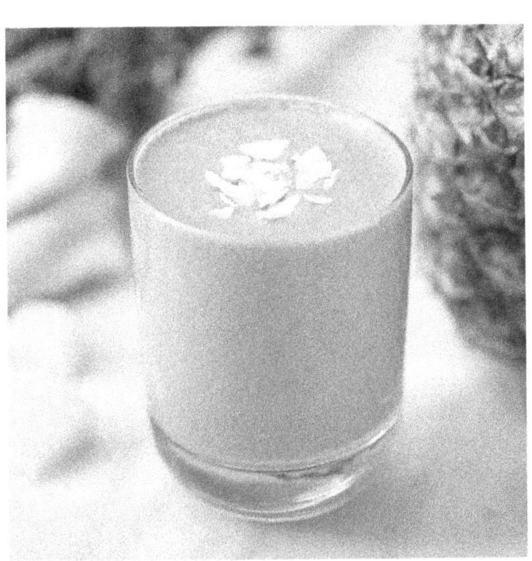

**<u>INGREDIENTS</u>** (for 1 serving)
Frozen broccoli – 1 cup
Pineapple – 1 cup
Banana – 1
Fresh baby spinach – 2 cups
Unsweetened almond milk – 240 ml

**<u>INSTRUCTIONS</u>**
1. Put peeled banana, frozen broccoli, pineapple slices, chopped spinach into your blender.
2. Pulse until smooth.
<u>Nutritional values (per 1 serving)</u>
Carbs – 74 g, protein – 9 g, energy – 339 kcal

## *31. Banana-Peanut Butter Green Smoothie Recipe with Broccoli*

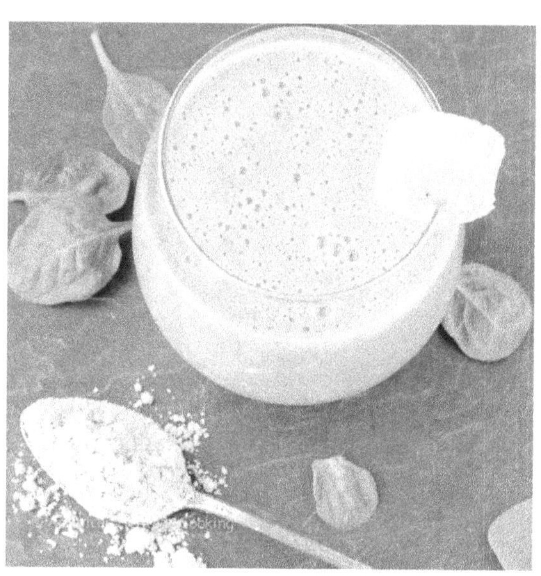

**<u>INGREDIENTS</u>** <u>(for 1 serving)</u>
Banana – 1piece
Frozen broccoli – 1 cup
Peanut butter – ½ tbsp
Baby spinach – ½ cup
Water – 225 ml

## <u>INSTRUCTIONS</u>
1. Put peeled banana, chopped frozen broccoli, peanut butter and baby spinach into a blender. Pour in water.
2. Blend well and enjoy!
<u>Nutritional values (per 1 serving)</u>
Carbs – 32 g, protein – 5 g, fat – 4,9 g, energy – 172 kcal

## 32. Basic Banana and Broccoli Smoothie

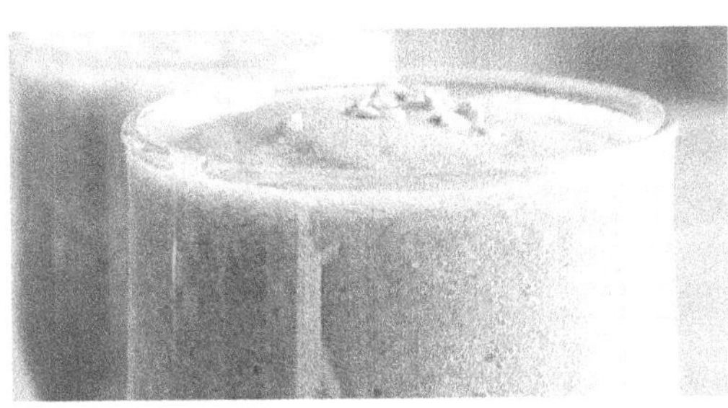

## INGREDIENTS (for 1 serving)

Bananas – 2 pcs
Frozen broccoli – 2 cups
Water – 225 ml

## INSTRUCTIONS

1. Combine peeled banana, chopped broccoli and water. Pulse well until smooth.
2. Enjoy!

Nutritional values (per 1 serving)
Carbs – 37 g, protein – 4 g, fat – 0,8 g, energy – 152 kcal

## *33. Broccoli Grapefruit Detox*

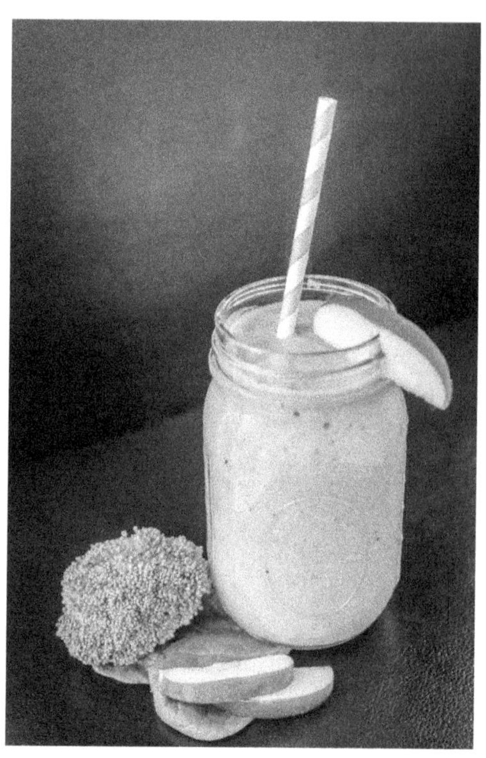

**INGREDIENTS** (for 1 serving)
Banana – 1 piece
Broccoli – 1 cup
Half of one red grapefruit
Homemade almond milk – 225 ml

**INSTRUCTIONS**
1. Combine peeled banana, peeled half of one red grapefruit, chopped broccoli and milk. Blend.
2. Taste it!
Nutritional values (per 1 serving)
Carbs – 55 g, protein – 7 g, fat – 4 g, energy – 264 kcal

## *34. SUPER GREEN SPIRULINA SMOOTHIE (5 INGREDIENTS!)*

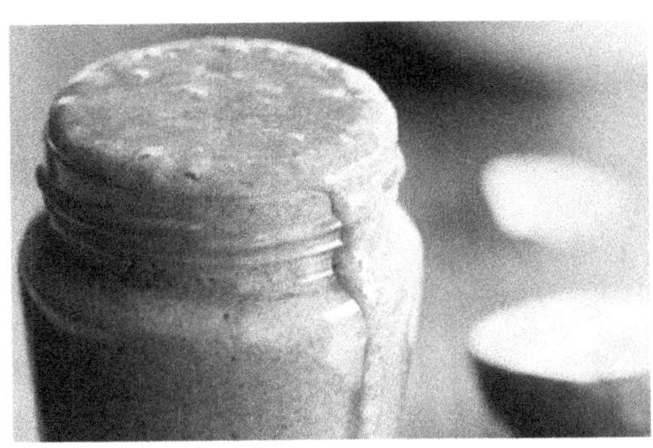

## INGREDIENTS (for 1 serving)
Frozen banana – 1 piece
Sliced cucumber – 50 gr
Coconut milk - 240 ml
Chopped kale  - 30 gr
Spirulina powder – 5 gr
Chia seeds – 10 gr

## INSTRUCTIONS
1. Throw peeled frozen banana, sliced cucumber, chopped kale in a blender. Add chia seeds, spirulina powder and pour in milk.
2. Blend until creamy and smooth.
3. You may keep smoothie keep in the fridge up to 2 days. Or freeze it and keep for 1 week.
4. Serve with fresh blueberries and granola.
Nutritional values (per 1 serving) – without toppings
Carbs – 36,8 g, protein – 5,8 g, fat – 4 g, sugar: 15.4 g, energy – 225 kcal

## *35. Apple Dandelion Green Smoothie Recipe*

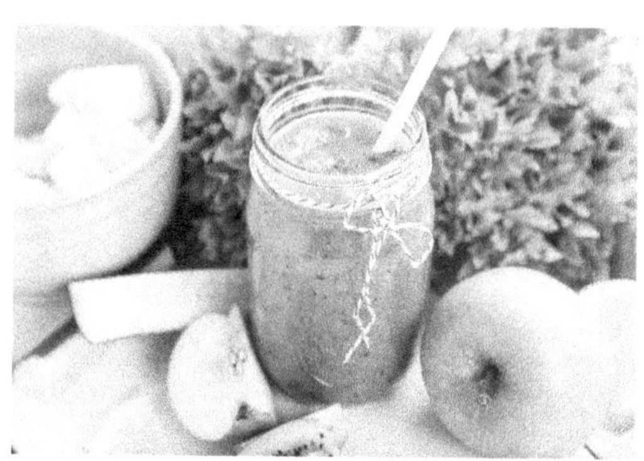

**INGREDIENTS** (for 1 serving)
Water – 240 ml
Apple – 1 piece
Frozen banana – 1 piece
Dandelion greens – 1 cup
Half of one lemon
The Add-ons
Chia seeds – 15 gr
Coconut flakes – 15 gr
Coconut oil – 10 ml
Green superfood powder – 1 serving

**INSTRUCTIONS**
1. Core and dice apple, peel and remove seeds from the lemon.
2. Put all necessary ingredients into the blender. Pulse for 30-45 until smooth.
Nutritional values (per 1 serving)
Carbs – 59 g, protein – 3 g, fat – 1 g, fiber – 10 g, sugar - 34 g, energy – 230 kcal

## *36. Ginger Detox Twist*

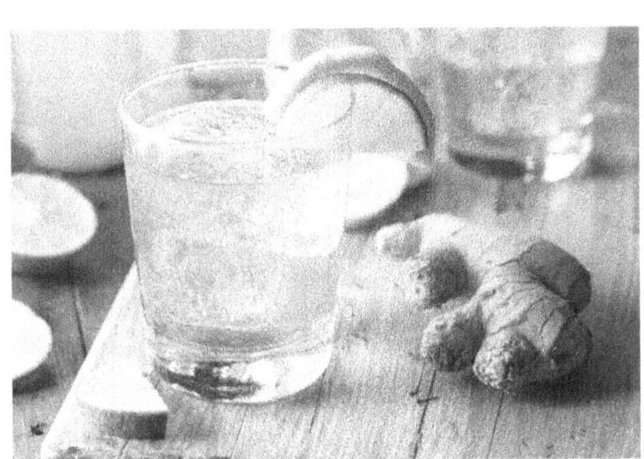

## <u>INGREDIENTS</u> (for 2 servings)

Collard greens – 1,5 cup
Persian cucumbers – 2 pcs    - chopped1
Apple – 1 piece
Meyer lemon – 1 piece   – peeled
Ginger – to taste
Chlorella – ½ tsp
Water – 240 ml
Ice – 1cup

## <u>INSTRUCTIONS</u>
1. Prepare fruits and veggies: peel lemon, chop cucumbers and dice apple.
2. Combine all necessary ingredients in your blender. Blend until desired consistency.
<u>Nutritional values (per 1 serving)</u>
Carbs – 22 g, protein – 5 g, fat – 1 g, energy – 114 kcal

### *37. Watermelon Dandelion Greens Detox Smoothie Recipe*

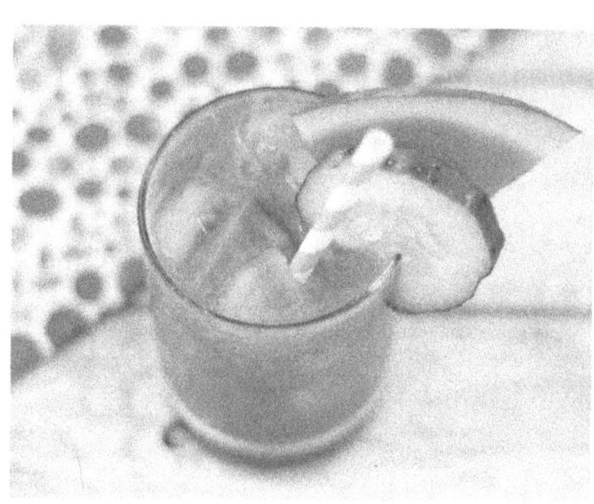

**INGREDIENTS** (for 1 serving)
Water – 120 ml
Fresh seeded watermelon – 1 cup
Frozen banana – 1 piece
Chopped dandelion greens – 1 cup
Juice from half of one lime
Cinnamon – 2 gr
Maple syrup – to taste
The Add-ons
Turmeric – 5 gr
Fresh grated ginger – 5 gr
Juice from half of one lemon

**INSTRUCTIONS**
1. Use high-speed blender. Combine all ingredients and blend until smooth.
2. Enjoy!
Nutritional values (per 1 serving)
Carbs – 45 g, protein – 4 g, fat – 1 g, fiber – 6 g, sugar – 25 g, energy – 182 kcal

## *38. Kiwi Pear Power Smoothie*

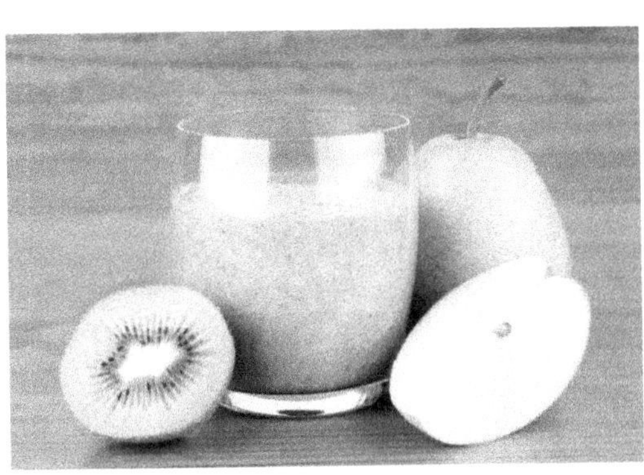

**INGREDIENTS** (for 2 servings)
Baby red Russian kale – 45 gr
Pear – 1 piece
Kiwi - 1 piece
Reishi mushroom – 1 tsp
Cashews – 45 gr
Coconut water – 240 ml
Ice – 1 cup

**INSTRUCTIONS**
1. Use high-speed blender. Combine all ingredients and blend until smooth.
2. Enjoy!
Nutritional values (per 1 serving)
Carbs – 30 g, protein – 3 g, fat – 7 g, energy – 183 kcal

## *39. Dill Detox*

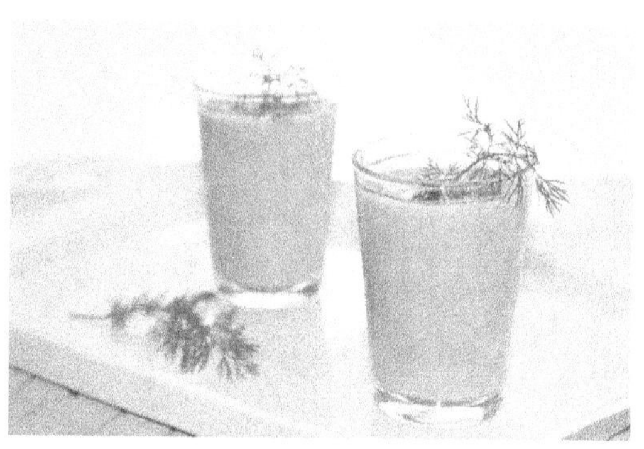

**INGREDIENTS** (for 2 servings)
Baby spinach – 45 gr
Persian cucumbers – 2 pcs
Pear –  1 piece
Fresh juice of one lime
Dill – 2 springs
Pomegranate powder – 5 gr
Water – 240 ml
Ice – 1 cup

**INSTRUCTIONS**
1. Chop pear. Combine all ingredients and blend until smooth.
2. Enjoy!
Nutritional values (per 1 serving)
Carbs – 22 g, protein – 1,4 g, fat – 0,3 g, fiber – 6 g, sugar – 8 gr, energy – 85 kcal

## *40. Mango, Banana and Spinach Smoothie*

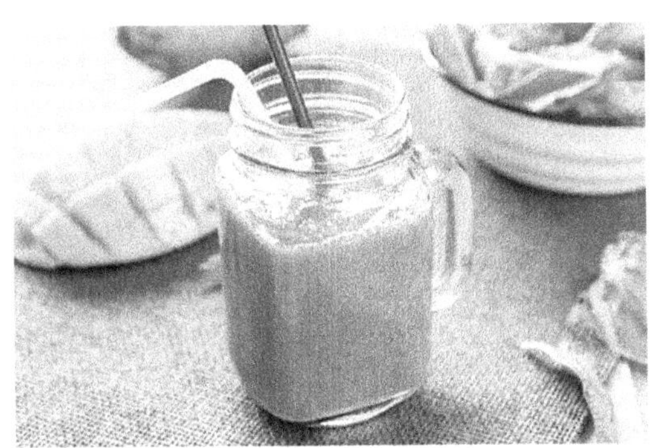

**<u>INGREDIENTS</u>** <u>(for 2 servings)</u>
Banana – 1 piece
Mango – 1 piece
Coconut milk – 120 ml
Spinach – 30 gr
Ginger to taste
<u>Optional Ingredients</u>
Vanilla protein powder – 1 tsp
Acai powder – 3 gr
Maca – 1 tsp
Chia seeds – 15 gr
Ice cubes

**<u>INSTRUCTIONS</u>**
1. Combine mango, banana and coconut milk. Blend well.
2. Add chopped spinach, ginger and blend again.
3. Add ice cubes and drizzle with chia seeds.
4. Enjoy!
<u>Nutritional values (per 120 g serving)</u>
Carbs – 27,6 g, protein – 1,3 g, fat – 0,4 g, energy – 106 kcal

## *41. New Year Detox Green Smoothie*

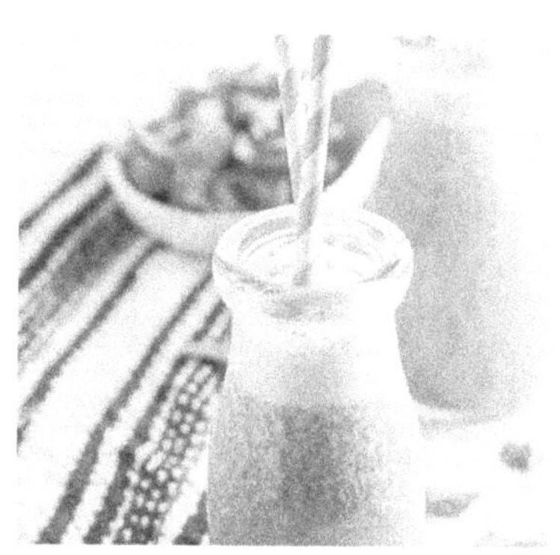

## **INGREDIENTS** (for 1 serving)
Frozen bananas – ½ cup
Green tea – 120 ml
Chopped mint – 15 gr
Spinach – 30 gr
Coconut water – 220 ml
Protein and Greens Vanilla protein powder – 1 scoop

## **INSTRUCTIONS**
1. Just put all smoothie ingredients into a blender.
2. Pulse until smooth.
3. Pour into glasses.
4. Add ice cubes and enjoy cold.

## *42. Orange Pineapple Green Smoothie*

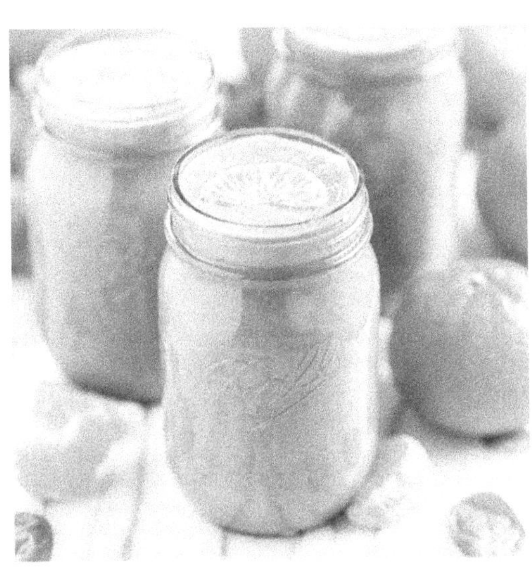

**INGREDIENTS** (for 2 servings)
Vanilla Greek yogurt – 240 ml (low-fat)
Water – 240 ml
Spinach – 60 gr
Orange – 1 piece
Banana – 1 piece
Pineapple – 1 cup
Ice

**INSTRUCTIONS**
1. Peel orange and banana, dice pineapple.
2. Just combine all smoothie ingredients in your blender.
3. Pulse until ready.
Nutritional values (per 1 serving)
Carbs – 55 g, protein – 13 g, fat – 2 g, energy – 273 kcal

## *43. Cucumber and Green Grape Smoothie*

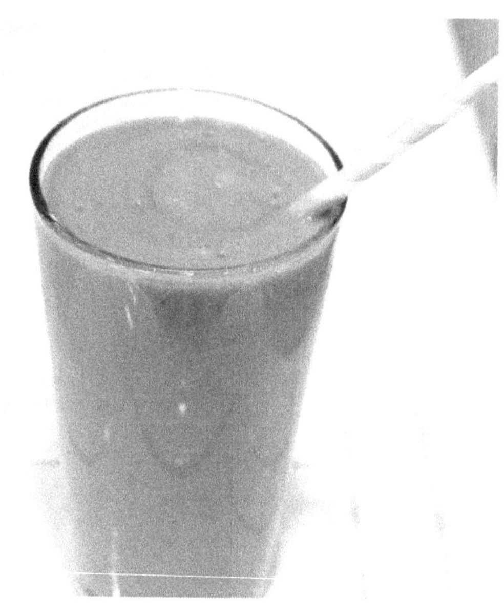

**INGREDIENTS** (for 2 servings)
Sweetened almond milk – 360 ml
Kirby cucumber – 1 piece
Green seedless grapes – 1 cup
Celery leaf – 2 stalks
Honey – 30 gr

**INSTRUCTIONS**
1. Peel and slice cucumber, peel and slice celery leaves.
2. Combine almond milk, peeled and sliced cucumber, frozen grapes, sliced celery, add honey and blend until smooth.
3. Pour into glasses. Enjoy!
Nutritional values (per 1 serving)
Carbs – 25 g, protein – 2 g, fat – 2 g, energy – 115 kcal

## *44. Mango Ginger Kale Smoothie*

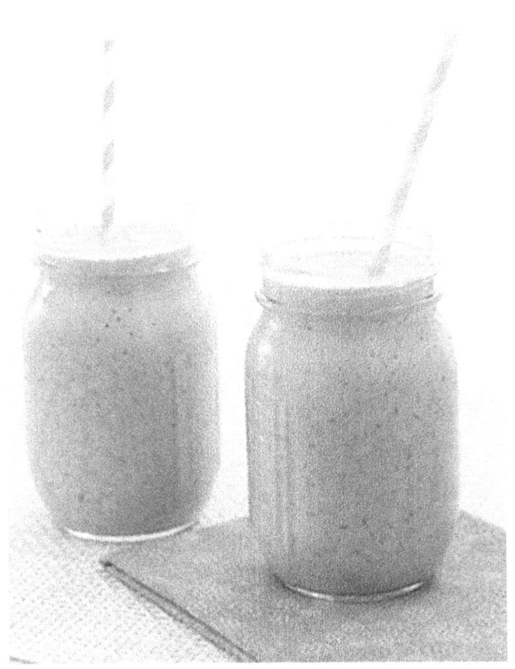

**INGREDIENTS** (for 2 servings)
Ice – 1 cup
Frozen kale – 60 gr
Frozen mango cubes – 165 gr
Frozen peaches – 150 gr
Fresh ginger – 6 gr
Lemons - 2 pcs
Water – 480 ml
Maple syrup – 15ml

## **INSTRUCTIONS**

1. Crush ice cubes. Then add frozen kale, mango cubes, peaches, fresh ginger, lemon juice. Blend.
2. Water and blend until smooth. Add syrup to taste.

<u>Nutritional values (per 1 serving)</u>

Carbs – 26,4 g, protein – 2,5 g, fat – 0,8 g, fiber – 3,5 g, sugar – 19 g, energy – 117 kcal

## *45. CREAMY SPINACH AND GINGER SMOOTHIE*

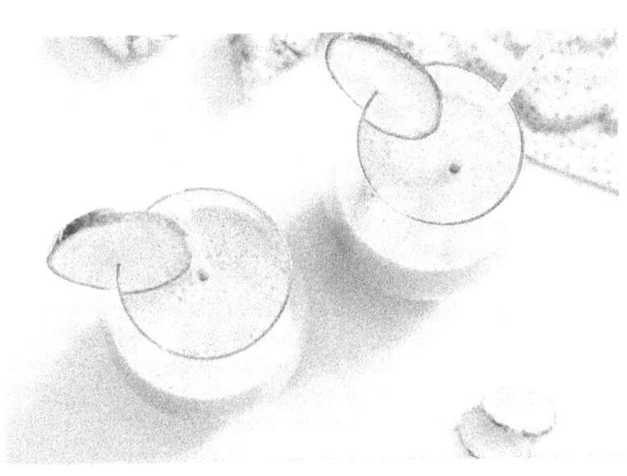

**INGREDIENTS** (for 2 servings)
Coconut milk – 200ml
Spinach – 60 gr
Ginger to taste
Banana -1 piece
Organic Burst spirulina tablets – 2 pcs
Organic Burst baobab powder – 10 gr
Avocado – 1 piece
Lime juice – 1 piece
Honey

**INSTRUCTIONS**
1. Combine all ingredients in a blender. Blend until smooth and creamy.
2. Enjoy!
Nutritional values (per 1 serving)
Carbs – 117,3 g, protein – 57,6 g, fat – 47,8 g, energy – 1032 kcal

## *46. Green Blast Smoothie*

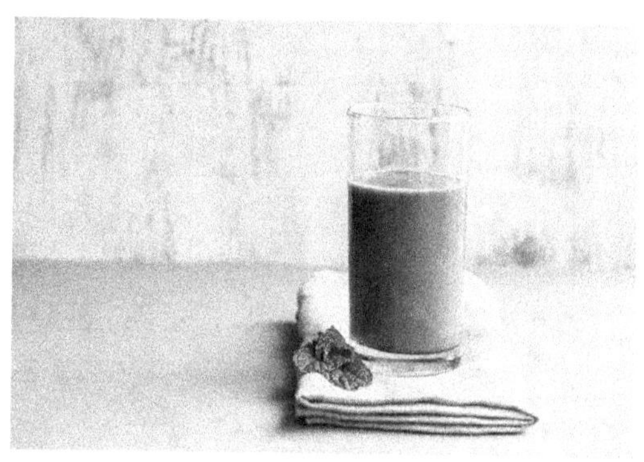

**<u>INGREDIENTS</u>** (for 1 serving)
Spinach – 30 gr
Parsley -15 gr
Mint leaves – 5 pcs
Cucumber – 1/2
Apple – 1 piece
SuperFood Fat Burning Boost – 15 gr
Coconut oil – 15 ml
Coconut water – 120 ml
Unsweetened almond milk – 240ml

## <u>INSTRUCTIONS</u>
1. Combine all ingredients in a blender. Blend until smooth and creamy.
2. Enjoy!
Nutritional values (per 1 serving)
Carbs – 39,0 g, protein – 5,1 g, fiber – 11,4 g, fat – 17,1 g, energy – 318,1 kcal

## *47. Skinny Green Tropical Smoothie*

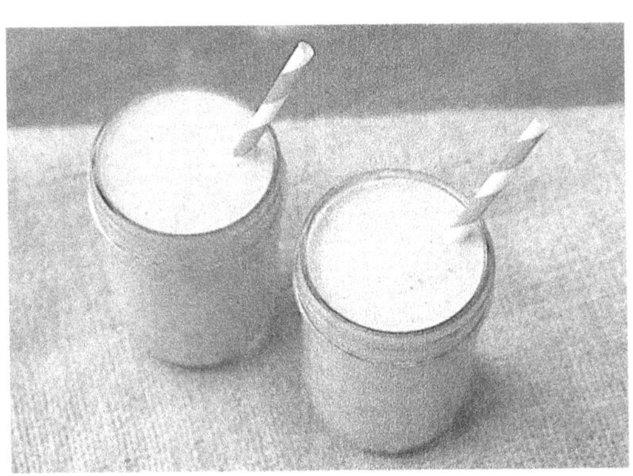

**INGREDIENTS** (for 2 servings)
Coconut milk – 180ml
Greek yogurt (fat free) – 180 ml
Fresh pineapple ¾ cup
Banana – 1 piece
Spinach – 30 gr
Sweetened shredded coconut – 30 gr
Ice

**INSTRUCTIONS**
1. Place everything into your blender.
2. Blend until smooth.
3. Drink cool!
Nutritional values (per 1 ¾ cups serving)
Carbs – 30,2 g, protein – 10,2 g, fat – 7,7 g, fiber – 3,9 g, sugar – 19,4 g, energy – 228 kcal

## *48. Pineapple & Kale Smoothie*

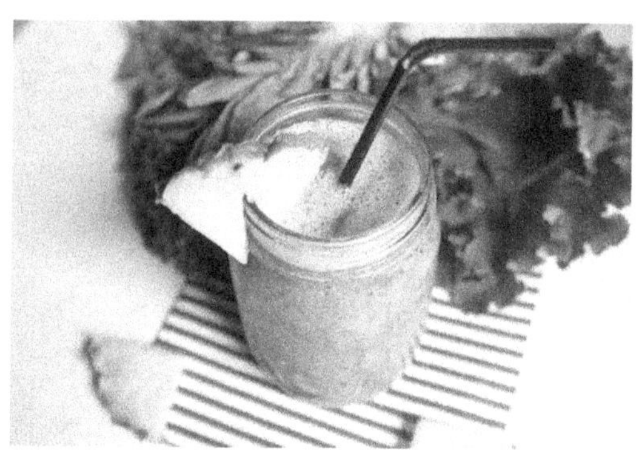

**INGREDIENTS** (for 1 serving)
Half of one pineapple
Kale – 1 handful
Coconut milk – 240 ml

**INSTRUCTIONS**
1. Blend chopped pineapple and coconut milk.
2. Add kale. Blend everything until smooth.
3. Drizzle with chia seeds. Enjoy!
Nutritional values (per 72,5 g serving)
Carbs – 13,6 g, protein – 2,1 g, fat – 2,2 g, energy – 79,5 kcal

## *49. Apple with Celery, Pear and Broccoli Smoothie*

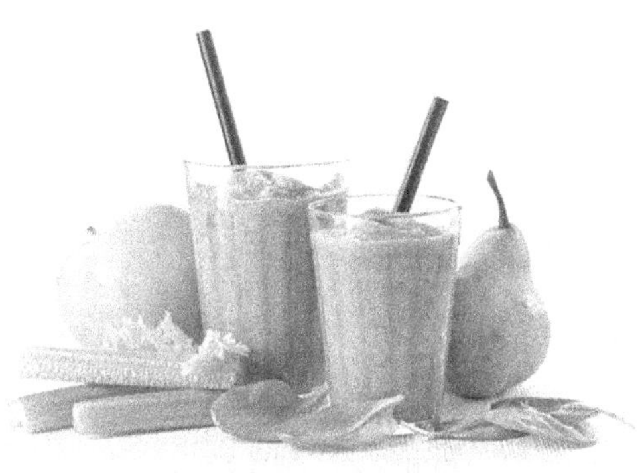

**INGREDIENTS** (for 1 serving)
Apple – 1 piece
Celery – 2 stalks
Pear – 1 piece
Broccoli – 2 crowns
Water – 180 ml

**INSTRUCTIONS**
1. Blend all ingredients until smooth.
2. Garnish with celery stalks.
Nutritional values (per 1 serving)
Carbs – 62,17 g, protein – 4,03 g, fat – 0,97 g, energy – 243 kcal

## *50. Coconut, Mango, Kale, and Lime Smoothie*

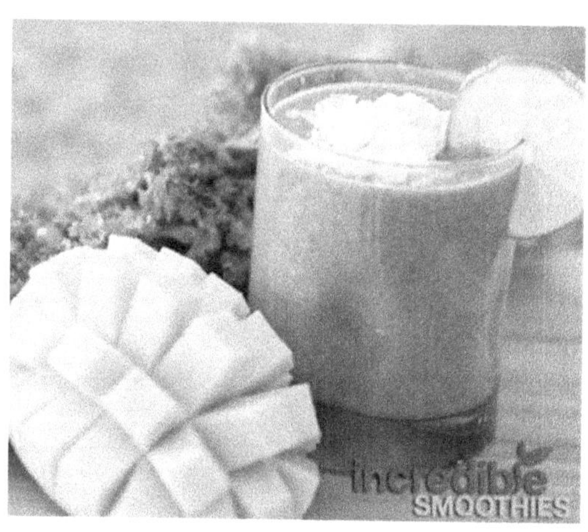

## <u>INGREDIENTS</u> (for 1 serving)
Mango – 1 piece
Half of one lime
Half of one banana
Kale – 90 gr
Unsweetened coconut milk – 225 ml

## <u>INSTRUCTIONS</u>
1. Peel lime and remove seeds, peel banana and slice it.
2. Firstly, blend coconut milk with soft fruit.
3. Then add harder fruits. Pulse until smooth.
<u>Nutritional values (per 1 serving)</u>
Carbs – 75 g, protein – 10 g, fat – 3 g, fiber – 10,5g, energy – 318 kcal